Intermittent Fasting

A Complete Beginners Guide to Intermittent Fasting For Weight Loss, Increased Energy, and A Healthy Life

PS: I Owe You!

Thank you for stopping by.

My name is Antony and I am passionate about teaching people literally everything I know about different aspects of life. I am an author and a ghostwriter. I run a small ghostwriting company with slightly over 100 writers. My wife (Faith) and I manage the business along with several other members of the team (editors).

Nice to meet you!

I started publishing (at Fantonpublishers.com) because I'd love to impart the knowledge I gather every single day in my line of work (reading and editing over 10 ghostwritten books every single day). My ghostwriting company deals with literally every topic under the sun, which puts me at a very unique position to learn more in a month than I learnt in my 4 years as a Bachelor of Commerce, Accounting, student. I am constantly answering questions from my friends, relatives and even strangers on various topics that I come across every day at work.

After several years of helping people to achieve different goals (e.g. weight loss, making money online, human resources, management, investing, stress reduction, depression, budgeting, saving etc.) offline thanks to my 'street' as well as 'class' knowledge on different topics, I realized I could be of better help to the world by publishing what I learn. My books are a reflection of what I have been gathering over the years. That's why they are not just focused on one niche but every niche possible out there.

If you would love to be part of my lovely audience who want to change multiple aspects of their life, subscribe to our newsletter http://bit.ly/2fantonpubnewbooks or follow us on social media to receive notifications whenever we publish new books on any niche. You can also send me an email; I would love to hear from you!

PS: Valuable content is my bread and butter. And since I have lots of it to go around, I can share it freely (not everything is about money - **changing lives comes first!**)

I promise; I am busy just as you are and won't spam (I hate spam too)!

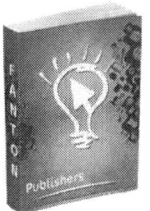

Antony,

Website: http://www.fantonpublishers.com/

Email: Support@fantonpublishers.com

Twitter: https://twitter.com/FantonPublisher

Facebook Page:
https://www.facebook.com/Fantonpublisher/

Private Facebook Group For Readers:
https://www.facebook.com/groups/FantonPublishers/

Pinterest: https://www.pinterest.com/fantonpublisher/

Some of the best things in life are free, right?

As a sign of good faith, I will start by giving out content that will help you to implement not only everything I teach in this book but in every other book I write. The content is about life transformation, presented in bit size pieces for easy implementation. I believe that without such a checklist, you are likely to have a hard time implementing anything in this book and any other thing you set out to do religiously and sticking to it for the long haul. It doesn't matter whether your goals relate to weight loss, relationships, personal finance, investing, personal development, improving communication in your family, your overall health, finances, improving your sex life, resolving issues in your relationship, fighting PMS successfully, investing, running a successful business, traveling etc. With a checklist like the one I will show you, you can bet that anything you do will seem a lot easier to implement until the end. This checklist will help you to start well and not lose steam along the way, until the very end. Therefore, even if you don't continue reading this book, at least read the one thing that will help you in every other aspect of your life.

Intermittent Fasting

Send me a message on support@fantonpublishers.com and I will send you my 5 Pillar Life Transformation Checklist.

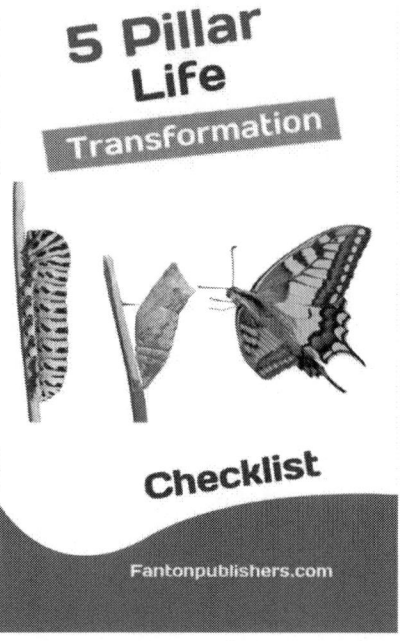

Your life will never be the same again (if you implement what's in this book), I promise.

Introduction

In the recent times, the gap between our meals has reduced to the point where we eat about five or even six meals per day (a mixture of main meals and snacking). This has brought so many problems that are unique to this era like obesity, diabetes, heart problems and so many other conditions, which are related to unnatural eating.

Why?

Our bodies were definitely not designed (or at least didn't evolve) to eat this way. In fact, this is not what will encourage optimal functioning in our systems but what actively destroys or undermines it. It goes against the nature of our body systems by loading it with all sorts of foods for longer hours and leaving very little gaps between the meals such that there is no time to clean itself up and derive energy optimally and efficiently from the food. This, according to me, is the worst injustice we do to ourselves. We get fat, drained, stressed and sick.

The solution lies in slowing things down and approaching eating the way our ancestors evolved to eat i.e. having one or two meals squeezed within a certain time window then taking the rest of the time off food to focus on other things. This is the essence of intermittent fasting and if you understand how it works and how to follow it then take action to follow intermittent fasting, you can be sure to benefit a lot. For instance, it can help you lose weight, burn fat, maintain a healthy body mass, keep you energetic, healthier and live a longer, happier life. This book will explain to you how that is possible, how it all works, and all the benefits you can reap from this pattern of eating and of course, how to start and do it successfully.

Note: While this book is designed for women (who are reportedly having the greatest challenge with weight gain and weight loss), even a man can read and benefit from it. Let's begin.

Table of Contents

PS: I Owe You!..2

Introduction 7

A Comprehensive Background To Intermittent Fasting.. 13

    What Is Intermittent Fasting?............................. 13

    Fasting Is A Natural Practice 14

    How Intermittent Fasting Works........................ 15

    IF and Women.. 17

    Intermittent Fasting Timelines 19

Benefits Of Intermittent Fasting 21

How To Undertake Intermittent Fasting 32

    Step 1: Understand And Select The Types Of Intermittent Fasting...32

    Step 2: Choose Your Foods Wisely 44

    Step 3: Breaking the Fast –Final Tips 51

Conclusion..53

Do You Like My Book & Approach To Publishing? 54

6 Things...54

1: First, I'd Love It If You Leave a Review of This Book on Amazon. 55

2: Check Out My Other Books 56

3: Let's Get In Touch 56

4: Grab Some Freebies On Your Way Out; Giving Is Receiving, Right? 57

5: Suggest Topics That You'd Love Me To Cover To Increase Your Knowledge Bank. 58

6: Subscribe To My Newsletter To Know When I Publish New Books. 58

My Other Books 59

    Weight Loss Books 59

    General Weight Loss Books 59

    Weight Loss Books On Specific Diets 60

    Ketogenic Diet Books 60

    Intermittent Fasting Books 60

    Any Other Diet 61

    Relationships Books 61

    Personal Development 62

    Personal Finance & Investing Books 62

Health & Fitness Books 63

Book Summaries 63

All The Other Niches 64

See You On The Other Side! 65

Stay With Me On My Journey To Making Passive Income Online 67

PSS: Let Me Also Help You Save Some Money! 69

Intermittent Fasting

© **Copyright 2018 by <u>Fantonpublishers.com</u> - All rights reserved.**

Let's start by building our understanding of what intermittent fasting is and what it is about so you know what you are getting yourself into.

A Comprehensive Background To Intermittent Fasting

What Is Intermittent Fasting?

Intermittent fasting (known as IF in short form) is a pattern of eating in which you eat and fast in a cycle. It mainly focuses on the time you are supposed to eat and rarely talks about the foods you need to eat.

This essentially means it is not exactly a diet, as in the traditional sense of a diet, that sets out what you should eat and how much you should eat. All it emphasizes on is that you should push your body to get to the fasted state by staying without food over at least a certain duration (normally 14-16 hours) then eating whatever you want to eat in the remaining 8-12 hours depending on how many hours you've been fasting.

What then does intermittent fasting aim to achieve through this? Well, the idea behind going without food for a minimum of about 14-16 hours is get the body into what's referred to as a fasted state, a state where it has already digested, absorbed and used up or stored all dietary energy molecules i.e. glucose (from carbohydrates), fatty acids (from fats) and amino acids (from proteins). During this time (the fasted state), your body is actively burning stored energy molecules i.e. glycogen from the liver and muscle cells and fats from different fat stores around the body. This entire process results to weight loss and a wide array of other benefits.

I know you might be wondering; how are you going to stay without putting anything that has calories in your mouth for more than 14 hours? Well, as I mentioned earlier, what we do these days is not exactly what is good for our bodies. In fact, it goes contrary to what our bodies evolved for over a million years to do. The idea of eating 3 to 6 meals per day and spreading them throughout the day such that the body hardly has any time to use what you've ingested fully is what is damaging our health.

Let me explain:

Fasting Is A Natural Practice

Basically, human beings have been fasting for millenniums, and particularly when there simply wasn't enough food available. This is one of the reasons why in the past, people were less likely to be obese, suffer from the 'modern' diseases like diabetes, obesity, brain disorders, cardiovascular diseases, cancers and so forth. Animals also instinctively fast when they are sick to heal faster and the process of eating and fasting (that is typical to the jungle setup) gives them energy and mental clarity to hunt efficiently even when there is very little to hunt.

My point is simply that there is nothing unusual or unnatural about fasting; and our bodies are perfectly equipped to handle long periods of not eating.

So how exactly does intermittent fasting work? Let's learn that.

How Intermittent Fasting Works

Let's begin with a basic understanding of how you gain weight to better understand how IF works to stop and correct that process.

When you eat a standard diet that is high in carbohydrates (this is the typical American diet that follows the USDA food pyramid), your body breaks down the carbohydrates into sugars/glucose, which is then absorbed into the bloodstream for transportation to different parts of the body. The glucose is meant to provide energy to the entire body. If the sugars (glucose) are in excess, because of eating too much of these carbohydrates, they first converted into glycogen within the liver then stored are stored in form of a molecule known as glycogen for later use. But since glycogen stores have a limited capacity, when the stores are full, the excess needs to be stored elsewhere. This 'elsewhere' is in fat stores around the body. To store excess glucose as fat, it is first converted into fatty acids and glycerol then transported in bloodstream as triglycerides to the fat stores. The entire process (uptake of glucose by the cells, signaling of the liver to make glycogen and fatty acids and glycerol) takes place with the help of insulin (a hormone produced by the pancreas). Insulin is produced in response to the rising concentrations of glucose so the more the glucose (because of taking more carb) the more insulin is produced to help clear the bloodstream of excessive amounts of glucose because these can be harmful to the cells if they stay there for a long period. Thus, the more you eat, the more insulin your body produces, and the more you gain fat- especially if you are eating a lot of carbs. Intermittent fasting puts break to the whole process of provision of glucose in the bloodstream. It also effectively starves the body of glucose and insulin, something that starts reversing the process that takes place when carb intake is high.

When you begin fasting, glycogen stores are typically the first source of fuel your body will turn to for energy- they are converted to glucose and put back into the bloodstream to be directly used as energy. When these stores have been depleted (as you continue fasting), the body turns to the fat previously stored in the fat cells for use in such dire circumstances. This way, all the fat you've been storing for years start getting broken down and being used for energy. Well, if you don't mind some science, this is what really happens in the burning of fat:

We have two processes on which your body's dependency increases as the glycogen stores are depleted:

- Lipolysis, where fat cells release the stored fat into the blood in molecules

- Oxidation, where the cells burn this stored fat

The body stimulates lipolysis through the production of hormones such as epinephrine, glucagon and the growth hormone (read more from the link below).

https://healthyliving.azcentral.com/mechanism-hormones-burn-fat-17398.html

These hormones enter your bloodstream and go to the fat cells and attach themselves to specific points referred to as receptors. In doing so, they release the fatty acids that are stored within.

IF and Women

You need to note that fat cells are not the same and don't usually respond well to the hormones. As a woman who has tried to lose weight before, you might have noted that certain areas of your body like the arms and upper body areas tone up but the belly and perhaps the hips being left unchanged. The reason this happens is that the fat cells normally have two opposing types of receptors for the hormones known as beta and alpha receptors.

The Beta and Alpha Receptors

The alpha receptors work to impede lipolysis while the beta receptors do the opposite. Thus, the fat cells that have a high amount of beta receptors are easy to mobilize while those that have a lot of alpha receptors actually make the process of burning fat harder.

The solution to this lies in finding a way to inhibit the alpha-2 receptors while keeping the beta-2 receptors active for efficient fat oxidation and fat loss. This is where the effects of intermittent fasting come in.

Note that when you begin intermittent fasting, your intake of insulin-spiking carbs generally reduces. Consequently, the insulin levels in your blood reduce and you get a double-whammy in favor of fat loss (since insulin essentially hinders mobilization of fat). Actually, experts place intermittent fasting alongside low carb diets as the most effective methods of inhibiting alpha-2 receptors because of their efficacy in reducing insulin. With low insulin, lipolysis can now occur better; thus, fat is broken down into fatty acids and glycerol and these products are then converted further into ketones and glucose respectively. Glycerol is converted into glucose through a process of gluconeogenesis and the fatty acids undergo a process known as ketogenesis to produce ketone bodies. As a consequence of ketogenesis, a ketone body known as acetoacetate is produced. This compound is in turn converted into two other smaller forms of ketone bodies called BHB (Beta-Hydroxybutyrate) and acetone. The former (which we're more interested with) is a more efficient source of fuel as it is used to supply energy to the body (after going through some more chemical reactions) including the brain. Actually, the brain and body have been seen to work better with BHB as a source of energy, and can use it with about a 70% more efficiency than glucose.

Therefore, intermittent fasting helps you lose weight and have the added advantage of having an energy boost throughout your body (you feel more energetic, are able to be more active and revitalized) all day.

Since intermittent fasting emphasizes a lot on fasting, it is important that I explain the timelines so you know how long you should fast and how long you are allowed to eat.

Intermittent Fasting Timelines

When you eat, it takes about 3-5 hours for your body to break down everything you've eaten into absorbable molecules and absorb it into the bloodstream for transportation to different parts of the body. Carbohydrates are broken into glucose, fats into fatty acids and proteins into amino acids. This period is referred to as the fed state and starts the moment you start eating.

By about 5 hours, all the amino acids, fatty acids and glucose from the last meal will already be in the bloodstream ready for uptake into the cells. Of note is the fact that the body relies on insulin to take up glucose into the cells (I mentioned this because glucose tends to be the biggest component of our food and the most problematic one because it contributes to weight gain if taken in excess- I already explained this). Throughout this period, the cells take up the glucose, amino acids and fatty acids through different metabolic processes. If there are any excesses, they somehow end up being stored in the body- glucose is first converted to glycogen then fatty acids if there is still more. It takes about 12-14 hours from the last meal for the body to use up or store everything in the bloodstream. This period is referred to as the post absorptive state and is often part of the fed state.

After the 12-14 hours have lapsed, the body then enters the fasted state, a state where it starts using up what it had stored. I already explained how the body breaks down glycogen- this happens with the help of glucagon, a hormone produced by the pancreas- and fats for energy.

From the explanation above, it is clear that for your fast to be effective, you have to dedicate at least 14-16 hours to get your body into the fasted state, as this will effectively enable you to burn stored energy. You can then schedule your eating for the remaining hours in the day. There are different approaches you can take to following intermittent fasting though including 5:2 diet, 24 hour fast, alternate day fasting, warrior diet etc., which we will discuss later in the book to help you to understand how to execute your fasts. For now, let's discuss what you stand to gain if you follow intermittent fasting.

Benefits Of Intermittent Fasting

Apart from what we've noted above, weight loss and increased energy, intermittent fasting does come with other benefits which include the following:

1: It Boosts The Immune System And Reduces Inflammation

If you've been researching about intermittent fasting, you should have come assertions about its efficacy in reducing inflammation, and as a powerful modality in increasing immunity and tissue healing as well.

What happens is that IF sort of flips a switch to trigger regeneration of the immune system, as it stimulates the body to produce fresh white blood cells. When you starve yourself, basically, your body system tries to save energy. In this case, one of the things it does to ensure this happens is recycle many immune cells that are not needed, particularly those that could be damaged (precisely why you'd notice many studies investigating prolonged fasting showing a low count in white blood cells as one of the noted effects). When you go back to eating, the blood cells come back.

The thing is; the depletion of white blood cells triggers stem-based regeneration of new cells in the immune system. A gene known as PKA shuts down and the stem cells go into regenerative mode. Think of it as the green light for the stem cells to start proliferating and rebuilding the whole system.

Perhaps you'd want to know that PKA has also been associated with aging, increased tumor growth and cancer.

Apart from that, intermittent fasting also controls the amount of inflammatory cytokines released in your body- some of the two major ones being Tumor Necrosis Factor Alpha and Interleukin-6. Both of these promote an inflammatory response in the body and fasting itself reduces their release to promote a stronger immune system.

If you are suffering from allergies and auto-immune diseases such as rheumatoid arthritis, systemic lupus, Crohn's disease and coalitis, the modulation of the immune system that comes with IF will go a long way to helping you manage the condition as the whole process eases the hyper inflammatory processes you go through and provide for a more normalized immune function. Looking at major diseases like cancer, you should note that the cancer cells have more insulin receptors than the normal cells- this is estimated to be between ten and seventy times more- and depend on glucose for fuel. As you know already, intermittent fasting reduces blood sugar and thus starves the cancer cells, leaving them weak and vulnerable to damage by free radicals and destruction in the long run.

2: Prevent Aging And Other Diseases Related To Oxidative Stress, And Promote Repair And Healing

You age because your body cells are actively becoming damaged by something called oxidative stress; thus, finding a way of preventing and repairing the cell damage resulting from the oxidative stress is thus a very helpful way to go against the aging process.

In case you're wondering, the stress we're referring to here is that which occurs when there is an increased production of free radicals than normal- such as oxygen reactive species. These essentially are unstable molecules that usually carry reactive electrons. The reaction is similar to that which occurs when something rusts- in this case, when your body cells are exposed to such reactions, they sort of 'rust'.

How it happens

When one of these free radicals comes across another molecule, it either gives up an electron or takes one from it. This can easily lead to a quick chain reaction involving giving up or taking away electrons between molecules, which forms more free radicals. The problem is that these can break connections between atoms inside vital cell components apart, such as the cellular membrane, the DNA or essential proteins. The obvious result is looking older quicker, and getting sick.

Just to put you into perspective, oxidative stress may lead to:

- Cancer

- Alzheimer's disease

- Neurodegeneration

- Diabetes
- Cardiovascular disease
- Cataracts
- Arthritis
- Autoimmune conditions
- Fatigue
- Brain fog
- Wrinkles
- Grey hair
- Worsening eyesight
- Depressed immunity

You need to note that free radicals can also be created as a result of the poor functioning of mitochondria (parts of cells that produce energy). When you switch between eating normally and fasting, the cells get a limited access to glucose and begin looking for energy in other sources like fatty acids- as you already know. As a result, the cells can switch on survival processes in order to remove the unhealthy mitochondria and over time, replace them with healthy ones, thus reducing the creation of free radicals.

Fasting also increases free radicals a bit early on during fasting and in response, the cells increase their levels of the natural anti-oxidants in order to fight against free radicals in future. Although the free radicals are usually seen as being harmful because they are able to damage cells, they could be vital short-term signals for your body in this case, stimulating the cells to cope with more severe stresses that could surface in future better.

NOTE: Many people also opt for external antioxidants to correct this process by transferring the required electrons in order to stabilize the free radicals before they bring about more harm to the body- I think fasting is easier because it is more natural!

The role of HGH

Intermittent fasting also boosts the levels of the human growth hormone (HGH), which in itself is a strong anti-aging effect, as it literally slows down the aging rate of your cells. When the HGH is released in your body, repair mechanisms automatically turn on. HGH mainly creates physiological changes in your body metabolism, which favors protein sparing and burning of fat. Your body uses the amino acids and proteins to repair tissue collagen, which boosts the functionality as well as strength of tendons, muscles, bones and ligaments. With good amounts of HGH flowing in your blood, your skin function is improved, wrinkles reduce, and any cuts and burns heal quicker.

3: Fasting Improves The Brain Function: Boosts Memory, Mental Clarity (Reduces Brain Fog) And Sharpness, And Supports Its Growth

To begin with, your endocrine system (the collection of glands that produce hormones) assists in balance and production of vital hormones thus assisting your body to grow and develop. However, your brain triggers the initial communication for the regulation of these hormones. The hypothalamus, which is the part of your brain that is known as the 'control center', basically scans the levels of your hormones many times each day. This part of the brain is in constant communication with the pituitary gland to ensure there is production of hormones from the thyroid, adrenal or parathyroid glands. The thyroid glands directly assist in regulating your metabolism. *Metabolism is the body's capacity to break down food and derive energy from it.* This gland achieves this by producing two types of hormones that regulate the system's function (T3/T4) both of which are in constant flux as a result of the signals being communicated by your brain. Your thyroid works in a feedback loop, and your brain keeps the metabolism running efficiently.

The problem comes in when you eat in excess (especially with most of the food being sugary or starchy), which increases your blood sugar very rapidly, or processed foods (which your brain could fail to recognize as instant fuel) can all affect the feedback loop to slow down your thyroid and brain (make them sluggish). This automatically leads to the slowing down of your metabolism, reduced mental performance and weight gain in the long run. Intermittent fasting ensures you eat less, increase insulin sensitivity by reducing the amounts of insulin in the blood and thus boosting your metabolism.

Memory and mental sharpness

1. As I mentioned earlier, IF boosts the levels of HGH in the blood which in this case assists in terms of neural processing, synaptic functioning boosting the memory and thought processing efficiency. There are studies (one done by intermountain medical center) that show that a mere 24-hour fast can boost your HGH circulation by 1,300 percent (for, men, the increase is about 2,000 percent).

2. With regards to brain fog, the main cause that has been identified is consuming too many sugars (usually due to eating too much food). Most people get the sudden rush and then fall into a state of fatigue. The main benefit of IF in this respect is helping your brain stop its reliance on glucose for energy and get the more sustainable energy from fats.

3. The brain's reaction to intermittent fasting has also been likened to that of exercising. The two activities affect increasing production of protein in the brain, which in itself promotes connection and growth of neurons while strengthening the synapses. *Synapses are the junctions*

between neurons that allow them to communicate properly with each other and keep the nervous system functioning the way it should. Intermittent fasting in particular stimulates the production of cells in the hippocampus, stimulates the creation of ketones and boosts the number of mitochondria within the neurons, which in turn assists the neurons keep their connections stable. All this has the overall effect of boosting memory as well as the ability to learn.

We could go on and on about the benefits of intermittent fasting on the brain, and how that would assist you in terms of leading a healthier, better life but with what we've seen so far, I think you get the idea:)

4: Improves Women's Reproductive Health and the Heart (Cardiovascular Health)

In the recent decades, it has become common knowledge that fasting helps in improving reproductive health and has been a common feature in reproductive health therapy. For one, certain health conditions related to the endocrine dysfunction that can negatively impact the reproductive health including obesity, Polycystic Ovarian Syndrome (PCOS), and metabolic syndrome can be improved or avoided by adopting intermittent fasting.

Most studies conducted on the subject have seen that women who suffer from PCOS tend to have reduced levels of stress neurohormone (*a neurohormone is a hormone produced by specialized nervous tissues instead of the endocrine glands*), which presents a positive effect on physical and mental health. They also experience a boost in the luteinizing hormone, which has a vital role in ensuring normal and healthy patterns of ovulation. This bodes well when it comes to balancing hormones, and is also a marker for fertility.

You however need to note that pregnant women are usually discouraged from undertaking any form of fasting but that doesn't mean you can't do it. If you are pregnant, you can tweak your food (on the feeding days). For instance, you can increase healthy fats and reduce or restrict the processed and refined grains during your pregnancy period. You can also consult your doctor to select the best method of intermittent fasting (see next chapter) to make sure everything is fine as regards to the pregnancy.

Note: most leading dieticians specialized in pregnancy and fertility are at the moment recommending a carefully designed diet that entails low carbohydrates and high fat for pregnant women that are suffering from gestational diabetes. With this, you don't have to understand rocket science to know just how useful (therapeutically) and safe these companion models of 'fasting' are.

How about the cardiovascular health?

You know cholesterol- the fat-like substance that is produced by the liver according to your body requirements- and which can also be acquired from food. Cholesterol moves around in your bloodstream in Low density lipoproteins (LDL) and High density lipoproteins (HDL). The LDL is also known as the bad cholesterol; it carries cholesterol to the areas of the body that require it but sometimes tends to cling on to the walls of your blood vessels (if you have too much of it in your blood stream), thus clogging them. That is dangerous because having narrowed or blocked arteries tends to prevent efficient blood flow to the heart, brain and other important organs. The result is heart attack, stroke, or even heart failure. Hundreds of studies such as the one below (which spanned eight weeks) have established that elevated LDL is a major risk factor for heart disease.

https://www.cambridge.org/core/services/aop-cambridge-core/content/view/S0007114516003445

The HDL on the other hand is known as the good cholesterol simply because it doesn't have the effects posed by the LDL, and because it picks up cholesterol then transports it to the liver to be disposed. Generally, to be in a healthy state, you need to have high levels of HDL and low LDL levels to assist reduce the risk of heart disease.

Intermittent fasting has also been proven by other studies to play a critical role in reducing LDL. In the 8-week long study below for instance, overweight and obese women fasting intermittently with one meal (500 to 600 kcal) on the fast days lost significant amounts of fat and their waist size reduced; they also had lower blood pressure, low blood glucose and of course, very low LDL (Low density lipoprotein).

https://www.ncbi.nlm.nih.gov/pmc/articles/PMC3598220/

Other studies have found the same improvements in cardiovascular risk factors regardless of whether people consumed a low fat diet or a standard American diet on the eating days. You can read more from the links below:

https://www.ncbi.nlm.nih.gov/pubmed/20300080

https://www.ncbi.nlm.nih.gov/pubmed/19793855

https://www.ncbi.nlm.nih.gov/pubmed/19375762

We have many more benefits of intermittent fasting that are beyond the scope of this book. The bottom line, however, is that intermittent fasting is the best natural deal you can get for healthier living.

Let's now see how you can put this eating pattern into practice.

How To Undertake Intermittent Fasting

Step 1: Understand And Select The Types Of Intermittent Fasting

Intermittent fasting is made up of many different methods, which entail different sizes of the *eating* and *fasting* windows. Today though, we'll focus on the best five methods, which have been proven and tested to be the most effective especially when it comes to weight loss.

The 16/8 Method Or The Leangains

This kind of fasting is ideal for someone who doesn't usually have time for breakfast.

The 16/8 is a method that proposes you fast for 16 hours per day and eat during the remaining eight hours (ideally two to three meals).

This method postulates that limiting your food intake to only eight hours per day is the ideal way and the easiest technique of weight loss and weight control. In this case, you have to eat all the calories for the day within this period- for instance, you can eat breakfast plus lunch at 10 am, lunch at 1 pm or 2 pm and then have your last meal by 6 pm.

In case you're wondering, the amount of calories or even fat that you consume within this period is not very important. The main argument behind this diet is that the typical long days we have, in which we eat food across as many as 16 hours is one of the main reasons most of us are having problems with weight management.

While the exact duration in which you can experience metabolic benefits from skipping meals is not known, experts say that going without food for at least 12 hours per day is beneficial- and going up to 16 hours is perfect. So, depending on your daily routine, you can choose when your eight hours will be. If you get hungry particularly in the morning, you can also decide to take breakfast as usual, have your lunch and then something very light by 6pm. This way, you will still have about 12-14 hours without any food every day, but are still consuming your calories so that you don't struggle with excessive hunger the entire evening.

Pros

The leangains diet is a great way to build lean muscle without putting on any fat. It has also been described as a great way to lose weight and be able to keep it off successfully. Unlike any other protocols of intermittent fasting, the leangains method entails eating every day; you'll not find any 24 hour fasting periods which means that the pattern essentially supports a rigorous schedule of training.

Cons

- The leangains method has a restricted time frame which has been identified as a problem because it tends to bring about the *dieting mindset*. This would make it difficult to follow the method for a long period of time because of the simple notion that it's a *diet*.

- Just like most other IF methods, the 16/8 method has been criticized for ignoring the theory of calories in/calories out which states that you are not supposed to eat more calories than you are burning off to lose weight (it gives too much freedom rather than limiting your calories on the non-fasting windows).

- Lastly, it is commonly held that leangains was built for bodybuilders in which case, some argue that the best results are only seen if you follow the protocol fully. This entails taking the right supplements at the right time with respect to the workouts and also very precise macronutrients and meal times.

Considering all the variables that the leangains diet involves, it can take time to work out the specifics of what would work for each person.

The 5:2 Diet -*Or Fast Diet*

This kind of fasting is idea for someone who needs a lot of flexibility.

The 5:2 diet is one that involves a restriction of calorie consumption to 25% of energy or calorie needs on two fasting days (non-consecutive) and eating ordinarily the rest of the week (five days).

Intermittent Fasting

During the fasting days, the total calories you should focus on as a woman is 500 (men should stick to about 600). You are free to choose when the two fasting days of the week will be; but just ensure you have at least one non-fasting day somewhere in between.

Theoretically, you eat normally on the non-fasting days and don't have to think about calorie restriction. This means that as you are generally eating less calories during the week, weight loss will be inevitable.

Tip: Most people who have reported to be successful with the diet usually plan their week in such a way that they fast on Mondays and Thursdays, where they consume two or three tiny meals and eat, as they would otherwise normally do on the remaining days.

Pros

- The intermittent diet is very flexible. The fact that you can choose the days you want to fast and the way you want to break up your calorie allowance (which can be between breakfast, lunch or dinner) means that the diet can fit into almost anyone's schedule.

- Secondly, the diet is not very limiting -like some fasting methods tend to be; it doesn't have any banned foods. Thus, it can mean being free to eat what you deem sensible without feeling limited to certain foods for five days per week. On the fasting days, however, you need to ensure every mouthful counts and that it is as nutritious as possible.

- Lastly, the two days that you are fasting also encourage you to incorporate more mindfulness around your meals as you plan them in order to eat the right amount of calories.

Cons

- A good number of nutritionists have questioned the sustainability of the diet and have argued that restricting calories severely for two days per week for your entire life may be difficult, particularly when you are eating out or over the holidays.

- Secondly, the 5:2 diet has a major problem when it comes to the eating days; telling people to eat whatever they like on the non-fasting days has been described as conceivably counterproductive to weight loss (one may take it as an opportunity to eat everything). In this regard, nutritionists have suggested that you understand that eating 'normally' is not a green light to eat anything. If you eat all sorts of unhealthy foods during your eating period, you can find yourself gaining weight instead of losing it.

- Lastly, when you stick to the low calorie limit required by the diet, it means not allowing for much food throughout the day, and this may lead to a possible elimination of essential food groups so that you achieve the strict

Intermittent Fasting

calories. In the end, you could find yourself eating poor quality foods overall as you try to limit your calories.

- This gets worse as you, like many people, find yourself fasting less and less owing to the flexibility of the diet.

The Warrior Diet

This method is ideal for someone willing to go the extra mile to lose weight

The warrior diet is an intermittent fasting method that entails under-eating during the day and eating a large meal (most of your calories) at the end of the day (dinner). The diet is based on a book: *The warrior diet* by Ori Holfmekler in which he describes the diet as having its roots in the ancient warrior nations. The Romans and Spartans, for instance, were very active physically during the day and could not have time to eat. They would feast at night when they were resting.

Implementing the concept behind the diet is simple: you only eat once, in the evening, which makes your fasting window about 20 hours long. The diet is flexible and doesn't focus so much on timing, or counting calories. Nonetheless, it has always been recommended that you choose healthy fats, large amounts of protein and vegetables so that you make the most of your fasting.

Like you'd expect, the diet does well in keeping you in the under-fed state during the day and inducing glycogen depletion really well. As a warrior, it goes without saying that exercising is important and should be done regularly. The warrior diet thus entails exercising sometime during the day- especially an hour or so before the meal. This makes fat burning even quicker and more effective. When you follow all that properly you'll be better able to use the food you eat in the body as you increasingly become more sensitive to insulin. This effect is actually greater than many IF methods would have.

Pros

- There fact that you are having one meal per day is good enough; no weighing, no lengthy planning processes, no weighing, major lifestyle changes or anything like that.

- Secondly, many people identify this method as the easiest plan with respect to schedule and food selection.

- Like I mentioned earlier, the warrior diet entails working out sessions. Therefore, the diet is able to assist in building strength besides shedding fat.

Cons

- One of the greatest concerns that has been identified concerning this diet is working out hungry, which can be tricky for most people. People claim that exercising while hungry can lead to muscle wasting, which can have an overall reverse effect. Moreover, your performance can reduce as a result of not eating before your workout.

- While these claims are valid, experts note that the statements are not necessarily accurate. These issues are less prevalent if folks on the diet get properly adapted to a strategy of healthy eating that includes eating high quality, natural proteins, fibrous carbs and healthy fats.

- Lastly, hunger has been singled out as a major concern as well especially affecting people who are just starting. If you are the type that typically begins feeling faint after skipping breakfast, the one meal per day may not be the most ideal method for you. Sticking with the diet requires you to be willing and able to tolerate a certain amount of hunger- initially at least.

The Eat Stop Eat method

The method is ideal for someone who doesn't mind some struggle mixed with flexibility

This program was founded by an avid weight trainer and nutritionist known as Brad Pilon. The Eat Stop Eat method basically requires you to fast once or two days twice per week (nonconsecutive); you choose 24 hours to fast and then resume eating the following day. In this case, you can choose to have your fast from 7pm to 7pm the following day so that you enjoy dinner before 7pm, and then wait to eat dinner after 7pm, making it simple to do the 24 hour fast. Now that you are free to choose the days you want to fast, the diet is thus very flexible; you can be able to work the days you fast around your personal program.

In case you have already began thinking that you cannot do it, consider that you already are fasting about 8-9 hours per day each night you sleep. It wouldn't be extremely difficult to stretch that a couple more hours, now would it? Let's assume you usually sleep at 9pm and wake up at 5 am. That's already 8 hours without eating.

Now add some 8 more hours to that; that's until 1pm. Now you've got a window between 1pm and 5pm to eat. You can begin with a light meal at 1pm and another light meal at 5pm to begin in the right direction before you are finally able to have one heavy meal to break the fast.

You have to note that just like the leangains protocol, the Eat Stop Eat is not your regular nutrition based plan for weight loss. It requires you to integrate strength exercises to build muscle tissue to assist you burn fat quicker -*note that even a little bit of muscle tone can assist burn more calories quicker and give you a desirable firm appearance.*

In this regard, the author of *Eat Stop Eat* (Brad Pilon) suggests you add some kind of resistance training strictly three times per week.

Pros

- You save a lot of money probably because you initially used to waste a lot of money on food (before you started fasting), and also because Eat Stop Eat will not ask you to purchase expensive foods but instead teach you why you don't need to spend so much on 'special foods'.

- Another major benefit of this method is that you don't have to stop going out with your friends (to restaurants and places like that) because the method is flexible (you can include light meals) and encourages you to lead a normal life as you lose weight.

Cons

- The method requires you to have self-discipline. While this method is a relatively new weight loss product whose guidelines are simple to follow and implement, you need to be committed to the whole thing if you are to see any real results.

- Secondly, the fact that you can eat anything you want has been overly criticized. This may make it feel liberating for you but as always, there's a very high chance you'll indulge in consuming unhealthy foods that could interfere with your weight loss goals.

- Lastly, hunger is inevitable- especially as you begin the program.

Other less popular methods of intermittent fasting include the following:

- OMAD (one meal a day) diet- entails taking one meal per day and macronutrient supplements

- Spontaneous meal skipping- entails skipping meals from time to time when you are busy or too lazy to cook

- Alternate-day fasting- entails simply fasting every other day

Your Choice

From what I have highlighted, you can select the type of intermittent fasting that you think would work best for you. Considering that you may only be starting, you can select two protocols, try them at separate times before you finally narrow down to the one you're most comfortable with.

You must have felt confused on the parts where the IF methods say you *can eat anything*, and then you get a suggestion saying that you need to *be careful with what you eat* or *stick to healthy foods*. There being no rules and the high flexibility that characterizes intermittent fasting protocols makes the whole thing attractive because you can eat things you love without feeling as though you are on a diet. This, however, can be a major setback when it comes to decision making because of the uncertainty you may experience when choosing foods.

In light of this, the next section briefly talks about what you need to eat and avoid during intermittent fasting, regardless of the method of fasting you're on.

Step 2: Choose Your Foods Wisely

To make the most of your calorie allowance on the fast day, you need to do the following:

Select meals that are higher in proteins. These foods will assist you feel full for longer. Protein sources usually have a high content of calories but all things considered, it still remains something worth sticking to. Let's take a few examples.

Grass-fed beef:

You get: (4 oz. strip steak) 26 g protein, 133 calories

Bison:

You get: (4 oz.) 23 g of protein, 166 calories

Ostrich:

You get: (4 oz. patty) 29 g protein, 194 calories

Pork:

You get: (4 oz.) 24 g protein, 124 calories

Halibut:

You get: (3 oz.) 16 g protein, 77 calories

Wild salmon:

You get: (3 oz.) 17 g protein, 121 calories

Light canned tuna:

You get: (3 oz.) 16 g protein, 73 calories

Pacific cod:

You get: (3 oz.) 15 g protein, 70 calories

Turkey:

You get: (Quarter-pound turkey burger) 16 g protein, 140 calories

Eggs:

You get: (1 egg) 7 g protein, 85 calories

Next, fill up your plate with low calorie, legumes or fibrous veggies. These will also fill your stomach for longer and provide you with other important nutrients like vitamins and minerals. You can steam them, stir-fry or even roast them in the oven with a teaspoon of oil and add a few pieces or flavorings to create a very delightful, filling meal. You can also have them raw in a large salad.

Here's a bit of what I'm talking about:

Artichokes:

You get: (1 medium vegetable) 60 calories, 4.2 g protein

Lentils:

You get: (1 cup) 230 calories, 18 g protein

Triticale:

You get: (1/4 cup) 161 calories, 6 grams of protein

Spinach:

You get: (1 cup, cooked), 41 calories, 5 grams of protein

Peas:

You get: (1 cup) 118 calories, 8 g protein

Ensure carbohydrates (especially the simple, processed or refined carbs) stay at the minimum. Besides being high in calories, they will easily make you feel hungry again. Some of the foods containing unhealthy carbs that you eat very infrequently or avoid include (but not limited to) the following:

- Parsnips
- White rice
- Pasta
- Bread
- Some fruits with high sugar (bananas, melon, grapes, dates, raisins, prunes and other dried fruits)
- Breakfast cereals
- Fruit juice
- Corn-on-the-cob/sweetcorn
- Cakes, cookies, candy, soda and other sugary snacks
- Anything else that is high in sugar like syrups

Don't be afraid of including healthy fat sources especially fish (examples highlighted above). While it may be high in calories, it will assist you remain full for longer. You can thus include little amounts of fat in your food before you fast.

In case you're wondering, ready-made meals don't have to be problematic at all. Just like the home-cooked meals, you only have to look for options that are particularly low in sugar and carbs and high in protein and veggies.

What to drink

Coffee and tea

Many experts recommend drinking ordinary tea a lot during intermittent fasting simply because it typically contains few calories and may not have a significant impact on your weight loss. This, however, would mean not adding sugar, milk or cream to your tea but drinking it plain- that's what I mean by 'ordinary'. Nonetheless, you can sporadically include artificial sweeteners if you find unsweetened tea unbearable.

How about the coffee? Well, you can take coffee during IF, but it should be black. That, according to me, means without sugar, cream or milk as they have calories. Again, you can use artificial sweeteners to flavor it if you want. Just ensure to avoid the coffee drinks in shops, as they are likely to contain some milk, sugary add-in or syrup.

Water

As you know already, IF takes many forms but most of them allow water. Actually, you should not go for very long without taking water. Besides other potential dangers, being dehydrated can cause unclear thinking, constipation, mood changes and kidney stones.

If you are on an IF method that involves some intake of food during the fast (for instance, some call for about 500 calories on the calorie restricted days per day) you could have about 9 cups of water (men need about 12 cups). Nonetheless, if your type of IF restricts food intake, you will get much of your hydration from plain old water. The general daily water recommendations from all the beverage and food sources are approximately 11 cups (for the men, 16 cups are pretty standard).

Low calorie liquids

First of all, you can consider fruit-infused water as it is not only hydrating, but also bound to keep your palate more interested on the fasting days. One of my favorites in this regard is water infused with oranges, mint and strawberries.

You can also look for unsweetened almond milk, which contains vitamin D and calcium- besides being very low in calories.

Lastly, you can make your low-calorie meals feel a bit more satisfying by adding warm, delicious clear broths. These can be vegetable, beef or chicken broths.

Step 3: Breaking the Fast – Final Tips

When you are ready to break the fast, you will first need to provide some instant energy to your body without experiencing a crash. Getting some *MCT oil* is a good place to start.

MCT oil is essentially converted into energy a lot quicker than other sources because it contains fatty acids that facilitate the production of many ketones more effectively than ordinary fat (long chain fatty acids) and much more easily. Thus, taking MCT oil will provide a lot of energy to revitalize your system before you start eating anything significant.

Next, you can also consider adding a bit of *apple cider vinegar* into the mix. ACV basically balances your pH levels, kills any bad bacteria present in your gut and most of all, stabilizes blood sugar, which you may direly need when you are coming out of a fast.

Hot lemon water is also great for this purpose because it contains citric acid, which supports the creation of digestive enzymes in your gut – this function is critical before you begin eating.

When you take these fluids, you are ready to transition to more solid foods such as unsweetened yoghurt and bone broths.

Next, start taking raw fruit and nuts, perhaps alongside vegetable juices as you transition into fully solid food.

Conclusion

We have come to the end of the book. Thank you for reading and congratulations for reading until the end.

If you never thought that intermittent fasting could be this simple, this beneficial and this good, I believe you now know better!

Now is your turn to take action!

If you found the book valuable, can you recommend it to others? One way to do that is to post a review on Amazon.

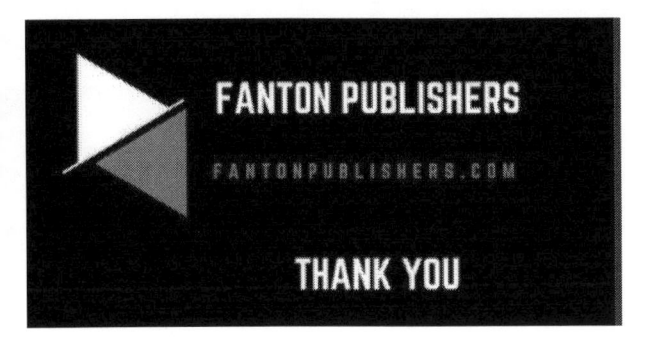

Do You Like My Book & Approach To Publishing?

If you like my writing and style and would love the ease of learning literally everything you can get your hands on from Fantonpublishers.com, I'd really need you to do me either of the following favors.

6 Things

I'll be honest; publishing books on what I learn in my line of work gives me satisfaction. But the biggest satisfaction that I can get as an author is knowing that I am influencing people's lives positively through the content I publish. Greater joy even comes from knowing that customers appreciate the great content that they have read in every book through giving feedback, subscribing to my newsletter, sending emails to tell me how transformative the content they read is, following me on social media and buying several of my books. That's why I am always seeking to engage my readers at a personal level to know them and for them to know me, not just as an author but as a person because we all want to belong. That's why I strive to use different channels to engage my readers so that I can ultimately build a cordial relationship with them for our mutual success i.e. I succeed as an author while at the same time my readers learn stuff that takes days and sometimes weeks to write, edit, format and publish in a matter of hours.

To build this relationship, I'd really appreciate if you could do any or all the following:

1: First, I'd Love It If You Leave a Review of This Book on Amazon.

Let me be honest; reviews play a monumental role in determining whether customers purchase different products online. From the thousands of other books that are on Amazon about the topic, you chose to read this one. I am grateful for that. I may not know why you read my book, especially until the end considering the fact that most readers don't read until the end. Perhaps you purchased this book after reading some of the reviews and were glued with reading the book because it was educative and engaging. Even if you didn't read it because of the positive reviews, perhaps you can make the next customer's purchasing decision a lot easier by posting a review of this book on Amazon!

I'd love it if you did that, as this would help me spread word out about my books and publishing business. The more the readers, the bigger a community we build and we all benefit! If you could leave your honest review of this book on Amazon, I'd be forever grateful (well, I am already grateful to you for purchasing the book and reading it until the end- I don't' take that for granted!). Please Leave a Review of This Book on Amazon.

2: Check Out My Other Books

As I stated earlier, my biggest joy in all this is building an audience that loves my approach to publishing and the amazing content I publish. I know every author has his/her style. Mine is publishing what I learn to readers out there so that they can learn what is trending, what other readers are also searching for in the nonfiction world and much more. As such, if you read the other books I have published, you will undoubtedly know a lot more than the average person on a diverse range of issues. And as you well know, knowledge is power- and the biggest investment that you can ever have on your life!

PS: If you want me to filter everything for you to include only Ketogenic diet books, you can subscribe to my newsletter and I will send you a list of all my Ketogenic diet books along with other useful content that I come across to ensure you succeed while at it http://bit.ly/2Cketodietfanton.

3: Let's Get In Touch

Let's get closer than just leaving reviews and buying my other books. Reach out to me through email, like or follow me on social media and let's interact. You will perhaps get to know stuff about me that will change your life in a way. As we interact, we will also influence each other in a way. I' definitely would love to learn something from you as we get to know each other.

Antony

Website: http://www.fantonpublishers.com/

Email: Support@fantonpublishers.com

Twitter: https://twitter.com/FantonPublisher

Facebook Page: https://www.facebook.com/Fantonpublisher/

My Ketogenic Diet Books Page: https://www.facebook.com/pg/Fast-Keto-Meals-336338180266944

Private Facebook Group For Readers: https://www.facebook.com/groups/FantonPublishers/

Pinterest: https://www.pinterest.com/fantonpublisher/

4: Grab Some Freebies On Your Way Out; Giving Is Receiving, Right?

I gave you 2 freebies at the start of the book, one on general life transformation and one about the Ketogenic diet. You are free to choose either or both!

Ketogenic Diet Freebie: http://bit.ly/2fantonpubketo

5 Pillar Life Transformation Checklist: http://bit.ly/2fantonfreebie

5: Suggest Topics That You'd Love Me To Cover To Increase Your Knowledge Bank. As I stated, I love feedback; any type of feedback- positive or negative. As such, make sure to reach out. I am looking forward to seeing your suggestions and insights on the topic. You could even suggest improvements to this book. Simply send me a message on Support@fantonpublishers.com. As a publisher, I strive to publish content that my readers are actively looking for. Therefore, your input is highly important.

6: Subscribe To My Newsletter To Know When I Publish New Books.

I already mentioned this earlier; I love to connect with my readers. This is just another avenue for me to connect to you. As such, if you would love to know whenever I publish new books and blog posts, subscribe to my newsletter at http://bit.ly/2fantonpubnewbooks. You will be the first to know whenever I have fresh content!

My Other Books

As I already mentioned, I write books on all manner of topics. In this part of the book, I have categorized them all for easy reading. If you wish to receive notifications about a certain category of books, I have provided a link below every category to ensure you only receive what you are looking for.

Weight Loss Books

You can search for the titles on Amazon.

General Weight Loss Books

The books in this category will help you lose weight irrespective of the approach you are using i.e. dieting or workout. I recommend you have them even if you are on specific diets or using specific workouts for weight loss.

[Binge Eating: Binge Eating Disorder Cure: Easy To Follow Tips For Eating Only What Your Body Needs](#)

[Lose Weight: Lose Weight Fast Naturally: How to Lose Weight Fast Without Having To Become a Gym Rat or Dieting Like a Maniac](#)

[Lose Weight: Lose Weight Permanently: Effective Strategies on How to Lose Weight Easily and Permanently](#)

Get updates when we publish any book about weight loss: http://bit.ly/2fantonweightlossbooks

Weight Loss Books On Specific Diets

Ketogenic Diet Books

KETOGENIC DIET: Keto Diet Made Easy: Beginners Guide on How to Burn Fat Fast With the Keto Diet (Including 100+ Recipes That You Can Prepare Within 20 Minutes)- New Edition

KETOGENIC DIET: Ketogenic Diet Recipes That You Can Prepare Using 7 Ingredients and Less in Less Than 30 Minutes

Ketogenic Diet: With A Sustainable Twist: Lose Weight Rapidly With Ketogenic Diet Recipes You Can Make Within 25 Minutes

Ketogenic Diet: Keto Diet Breakfast Recipes

Get updates when we publish any book on the Ketogenic diet: http://bit.ly/2fantonpubketo

Intermittent Fasting Books

Get updates when we publish any book on intermittent fasting: http://bit.ly/2fantonbooksIF

Any Other Diet

Get updates when we publish any book on any other diet that will help you to lose weight and keep it off: http://bit.ly/2fantonsdietbooks

Relationships Books

[Wedding: Budget Wedding: Wedding Planning On The Cheap (Master How To Plan A Dream Wedding On Budget)](#)

[How To Get Your Ex Back: Step By Step Formula On How To Get Your Ex Back And Keep Him/her For Good](#)

[SEX POSITIONS: Sex: Unleash The Tiger In You Using These 90-Day Sex Positions With Pictures](#)

[Money Problems: How To Solve Relationship Money Problems: Save Your Marriage By Learning How To Fix All Your Money Problems And Save Your Relationship](#)

[Family Communication: A Simple Powerful Communication Strategy to Transform Your Relationship with Your Kids and Enjoy Being a Parent Again](#)

Get updates when we publish any book that will help you improve on your personal and professional relationships: http://bit.ly/2fantonsrelations

Personal Development

[Body Language: Master Body Language: A Practical Guide to Understanding Nonverbal Communication and Improving Your Relationships](#)

[Subconscious Mind: Tame, Reprogram & Control Your Subconscious Mind To Transform Your Life](#)

Get updates when we publish any book that will help you become a better person by boosting your productivity, achieving more of your goals, beating procrastination, breaking bad habits, forming new habits, beat stress, building your self-esteem and confidence and much more: http://bit.ly/2fantonpubpersonaldevl

Personal Finance & Investing Books

[Real Estate: Rental Property Investment Guide: How To Buy & Manage Rental Property For Profits](#)

[MONEY: Make Money Online: 150+ Real Ways to Make Real Money Online (Plus 50 Bonus Tips to Guarantee Your Success)](#)

[Money: How To Make Money Online: Make Money Online In 101 Ways](#)

Get updates when we publish any book that will help you up your game in personal finance and investing: http://bit.ly/2fantonpersfinbooks

Health & Fitness Books

PMS CURE: Easy To Follow Home Remedies For PMS & PMDD

Testosterone: How to Boost Your Testosterone Levels in 15 Different Ways Naturally

Hair Loss: How to Stop Hair Loss: Actionable Steps to Stop Hair Loss (Hair Loss Cure, Hair Care, Natural Hair Loss Cures)

Hashimoto's: Hashimoto's Cookbook: Eliminate Toxins and Restore Thyroid Health through Diet In 1 Month

Get updates when we publish any book that will help you up your game in health and fitness: http://bit.ly/2fantonhealthnfit

Book Summaries

This category will feature summaries of some of your favorite books, written in a manner you can easily digest and follow:

Summary: The Millionaire Next Door: The Surprising Secrets of America's Wealthy

Get updates whenever we publish new book summaries: http://bit.ly/2fantons

All The Other Niches

This category of books includes anything that we cannot realistically fit in the categories above. As always, if you want just about anything you can get to read, this is the category for you!

Travel Books

[Kenya: Travel Guide: The Traveler's Guide to Make The Most Out of Your Trip to Kenya (Kenya Tourists Guide)](#)

Dog Training

[Dog Tricks: 15 Tricks You Must Teach Your Dog before Anything Else](#)

World Issues Books

[ISIS/ISIL: The Rise and Rise of the Islamic State: A Comprehensive Guide on ISIS & ISIL](#)

Get notifications when we publish books on anything else above from the niches I mentioned above: http://bit.ly/2fantonpubnewbooks

See You On The Other Side!

See, I publish books on just about any topic imaginable!

If you have any suggestions on topics you would want me to cover, feel free to get in touch:

Website: http://www.fantonpublishers.com/

Email: Support@fantonpublishers.com

Twitter: https://twitter.com/FantonPublisher

My Ketogenic Diet Books Page: https://www.facebook.com/pg/Fast-Keto-Meals-336338180266944

Facebook Page: https://www.facebook.com/Fantonpublisher/

Private Facebook Group For Readers: https://www.facebook.com/groups/FantonPublishers/

Pinterest: https://www.pinterest.com/fantonpublisher/

PS: You can subscribe to my mailing list to know when I publish new books:

Hey! This is not the entire list! You can check an updated list of all my books on:

My Author Central: amazon.com/author/fantonpublishers

My Website: http://www.fantonpublishers.com

Stay With Me On My Journey To Making Passive Income Online

I have to admit; my writing business makes several six figures a year in profits (after paying ourselves salaries). Until recently, I didn't realize just how hard we worked to build this business to what it has become so far.

However, while it is profitable and I want to do it in the long term, I understand its limitations. I know I cannot have an endless number of writers at a time especially if we are to continue delivering high quality products to our customers and readers consistently.

That's why I have recently started getting more serious with self-publishing to help me build a passive income business i.e. income that is not pegged on the number of writers and hours that we put to develop our products.

Thanks to my vast experience and dedication to get things done, I am committed to building a six figure passive income publishing business.

To make sure you are part of this journey, I am inviting you to [subscribe to our newsletter](http://bit.ly/2fanton6figprogress) to know my progress as far as passive income generation is concerned. That's not all; if making passive income, just like me, is something you'd love to venture into, you can follow my 'tell it all' blog, which I explain everything I have done to promote every book and how the results are turning out with figures and images.

My goal is to make sure that while I add value to my audience through the different topics that I publish about to solve various problems for instance, I also add massive value to readers in ways that go beyond just one book. Subscribe to our newsletter to know when I publish new books, how I did market research, how I make money with the books and much, much more.

You can even ask questions on anything you want me to answer regarding publishing and everything else related to the topics of discussion.

Antony

Website: http://www.fantonpublishers.com/

Email: Support@fantonpublishers.com

Twitter: https://twitter.com/FantonPublisher

Facebook Page: https://www.facebook.com/Fantonpublisher/

My Ketogenic Diet Books Page: https://www.facebook.com/pg/Fast-Keto-Meals-336338180266944

Private Facebook Group For Readers: https://www.facebook.com/groups/FantonPublishers/

Pinterest: https://www.pinterest.com/fantonpublisher/

I look forward to hearing from you!

PSS: Let Me Also Help You Save Some Money!

If you are a heavy reader, have you considered subscribing to Kindle Unlimited? You can read this and millions of other books for just $9.99 a month)! You can check it out by searching for Kindle Unlimited on Amazon!

Made in the USA
Middletown, DE
02 February 2019